THE CHUBBY YOGI

Antonio El Rico

Note: Although the author has made every effort to ensure that the information in this book is correct, the author does not assume and hereby disclaims any liability to any party for any loss, damage, or disruption caused by use and application of any of the contents of this book. Any resemblance to actual persons, living or dead, is purely coincidental.

Contents

Chapter 3: The Yoga Master   99

Chapter 4: Here's Some Workouts   119

Epilogue   128

Introduction

Congratulations, you somehow got your greasy fingers on this little book. What is it all about? This is a short, light-hearted, illustrated introduction to yoga. For everyone who is kind of interested in yoga but has the attention span of a goldfish. Or perhaps you don't like people and you want to practice on your own instead of in a class. Or maybe you're too broke for classes. It's also for people who may have no interest in yoga because they detest chanting mantras and have no interest in opening their heart chakra. Perhaps this book can convince you that you don't need all that stuff and you can still have a proper workout doing yoga, at all levels of personal fitness. Yoga is also a great stress buster, because you're combining deep breathing with working out the body. Whether you want to get fitter, skinnier, buffer, more flexible, stress-free, or all of the above, yoga can help you with that. There's really no excuse for not trying it. And if you do have excuses, just have a laugh at the silly illustrations.

How to use this book

This book contains more than fifty yoga poses for you to try, divided in three chapters based on difficulty. I suggest you start from the beginning, and only move on to the harder poses if you can do the easier ones without hurting yourself. As far as combining poses into sequences goes, do whatever you want. You can follow the order of the book, or you can pick the poses that improve posture, or those that stretch your hamstrings, or just pick your favorites. If you are completely clueless, the last chapter consists of some entry-level sequence suggestions.

In any case, it's always smart to warm up and stretch a little before you go at it. Always work within a pain-free range and consult with your doctor first if you have any medical conditions. You should challenge yourself, but back off if anything hurts before you strain something. Make use of any help if you can't do the poses on your own, whether that'd be a wall, a partner, a chair, your dog, or a yoga block. Speaking of yoga equipment, a yoga mat is a cheap purchase that, while not absolutely necessary, makes practice easier and more comfortable. Comfortable, stretchy clothes are recommended, or you can practice naked.

As for the practice itself, it's important to keep breathing during the poses. Breathe deeply while getting into them and while getting out. When you're in a pose, try to hold it for at least five deep breaths. Breathe vocally, that is, you should be able to hear your own breath. Many poses are beneficial when held for a longer period of time, so if you want to do a handstand for 5 minutes, feel free. Furthermore, the instructions in this book are compact, so if there's something you don't get, by all means, watch a Youtube video. And of course, getting a professional yoga teacher is always the best way to perfect your poses, though they will likely urge you to chant mantras and open your chakras as well. They will also charge you a shitload of money to sit in a hot room that smells like sweat and farts (due to opening the root chakra, maybe?). On the other hand, they do play relaxing music sometimes and you get to drink ginger tea with fellow hot yogis, so it's up to you, dear reader.

Finally, every single pose in this book has the Sanskrit name right next to it at the top of the page, so I suggest you learn these by heart and use them to impress your friends, if you have any.

"What are you doing, Patricia?"

"Just some Utthita Hasta Padangustasana."

"That's cool."

Chapter 1: The Beginner

Here we go, young yogi. A life-changing experience awaits you. And if you suck at it at first, remember this quote by some famous master:

"Yoga is 99% practice and 1% theory."

– Sri Krishna Pattabhi Jois

1. Mountain Pose – *Tadasana*

How to do it:

Not much of a pose if you ask me, but yoga masters will probably disagree. It is the starting position for other standing poses, so I will include it here as the very first pose. So how on earth do I do this, you're asking. To start, stand on your feet with your big toes touching. Hands by your sides, or in prayer position if you want to include some chanting. Stand straight, aim your tailbone at your heels and keep your chest forward but don't overdo it. You can try to rock the hips forwards and backwards a little to find your neutral position. Five deep breaths and move along. You can close your eyes if you want a bit of an extra challenge.

Why do it:

- The first step to becoming a yoga master.
- Improves posture and balance, this is how you're supposed to stand.
- Standing is healthier than sitting.

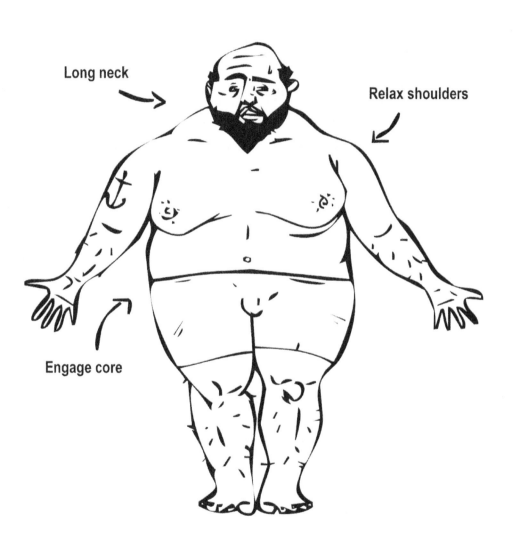

Long neck

Relax shoulders

Engage core

2. Easy Pose – *Sukhasana*

How to do it:

The name checks out, this one is pretty easy. To start, sit your butt down on a support (such as a blanket, block or cushion) and cross your legs such that your knees are lower than your hips. Bring the knees towards each other so that the feet are under the knees. Straighten your spine, chest up and put your hands on your knees or in prayer position. Alternate the cross of your legs every now and then. That's it. Breathe in and out until you attain nirvana, or until you're ready to move on to the next pose.

Why do it:

- It's easy.
- Good for your posture.
- Stretches the knees and ankles.

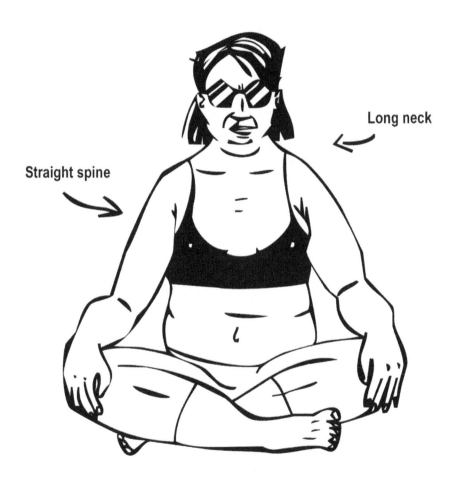

Long neck

Straight spine

3. Child's Pose – *Balasana*

How to do it:

This is a resting pose, in case you're already tired from the last two (or any other pose), but you're also stretching, so it's a good pose to get in the mood. First, kneel. Sit down on your heels and keep your big toes touching, but not your knees. Knees should be wide enough for you to drop your torso in between. Lower down and rest your forehead on the mat and your belly on your thighs. Arms may rest by your side, palms up, or you can place them in front of you for an additional shoulder and upper back stretch.

Why do it:

- Relaxes body and mind.
- Stretches hips, thighs, and ankles.
- As well as the shoulders and upper back (in the variation).

Lengthen the spine

Long neck

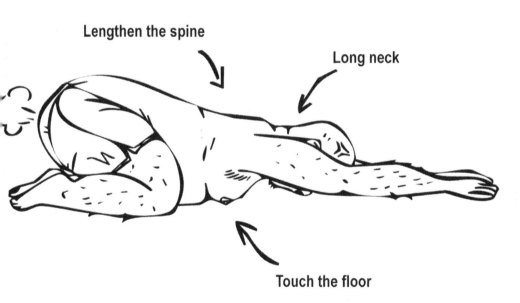

Touch the floor

4. Sphinx Pose – *Salamba Bhujangasana*

How to do it:

This one is the easiest of the backbends, poses that counter that forward hunch you have because you're sitting in front of a screen all day. This is also the pose of the majestic mythical creature with the body of a lion and head of a human. Or the naked cat breed, if you're into that. To start, get on your belly. Straighten your legs and walk your hands forward in front of you. Keep your elbows under your shoulders and your hands shoulder-width apart. On the inbreath, push and lift your chest and head upwards. You should feel the chest and abs stretching. Breathe in and out for five or until you feel like doing something else.

Why do it:

- Strengthens spine.
- Stretches chest, shoulders and abdomen.
- Relaxes body and mind.

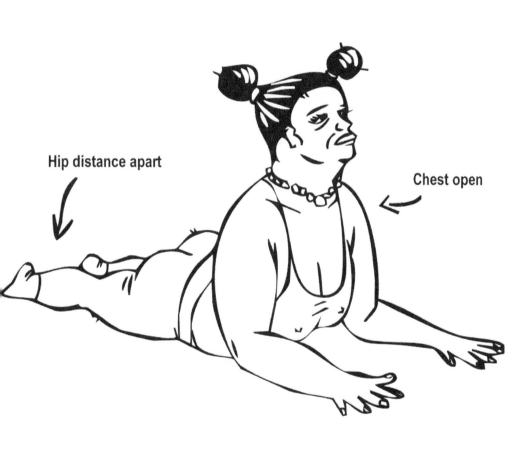

Hip distance apart

Chest open

5. Staff Pose – *Dandasana*

How to do it:

This may look easy, and it is. Sit on your mat and stretch your legs out in front of you. Toes up, straighten your back and place your hands next to your hips. With the help of your arms you lengthen your spine and point the crown of your head towards the sky while pressing your sitting bones into the mat. If you have a large butt, you may want to move your ass-cheeks out of the way a little for a more grounded feel. This is the starting position for many of the sitting poses, so get comfortable with it.

Why do it:

- Good for your posture.
- Strengthens the back muscles.
- Stretches chest, shoulders, spine and hamstrings.

Straight spine

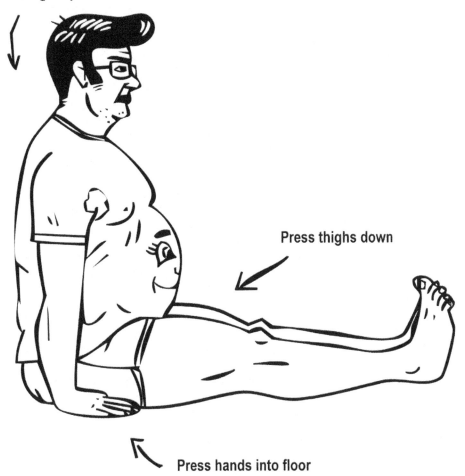

Press thighs down

Press hands into floor

6. Seated Forward Bend – *Paschimottanasana*

How to do it:

If you're still in **Staff** pose, good. If not, get into it. Sit down and extend your legs out in front of you. Keep your back straight and your toes up. Now lift your hands over your head, chin up and chest out, then fold forward as far as you can without hurting yourself. Hinge from the hips, not from the waist. Ideally, you rest your head on your shins and you catch your big toes with your index and middle finger, or you catch your wrist behind your feet for the greatest stretch. Realistically, you're probably not getting that far anytime soon, so just do your best. You may bend your knees a little if you're stiff as a board.

Why do it:

- Stretches spine, shoulders and hamstrings especially.
- Quite relaxing.
- Tradition says it can prevent or cure diabetes (don't ask me).

Flex toes

Hinge from hips

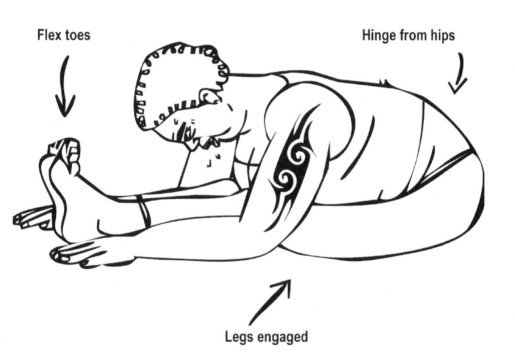

Legs engaged

7. Wide-Angle Seated Forward Bend – *Upavistha Konasana*

How to do it:

A variation of the previous pose. Start by sitting in **Staff** pose. Extend your legs in front of you and open your legs to about a 90-degree angle, or as wide as you can. Point up your toes and bend the upper body forward, hinging from the hips. Walk your hands forward as far as you can for a nice stretch. Perhaps you can rest on your elbows, or even bring your face or chest to the mat while your arms are stretched in front of you. If not, just rest on your hands and breathe in and out for five.

Why do it:

- Stretches insides and backs of the legs.
- Strengthens the spine.
- Opens the hips, groins and prepares you for childbirth.

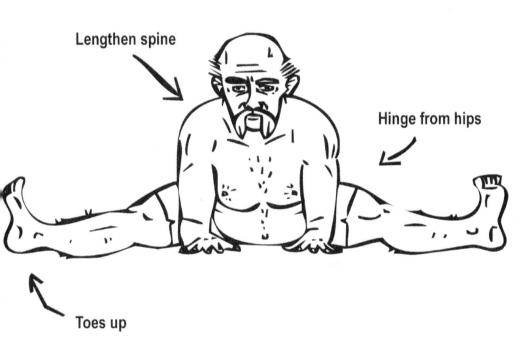

Lengthen spine

Hinge from hips

Toes up

8. Cow Pose – *Bitilasana*

How to do it:

Crawl on your hands and knees. Arms and legs should be perpendicular to the floor, with the knees right under your hips. Wrists, elbows and shoulders are in a straight line. You're a table. Inhale and drop your belly towards the mat while lifting your chest up. You're a cow now. Stay in the pose for a couple breaths or alternatively transform into a table and a cow with each inhale and outbreath.

Why do it:

- Stretches front torso and neck.
- Massages the spine and belly organs.
- You're a cow.

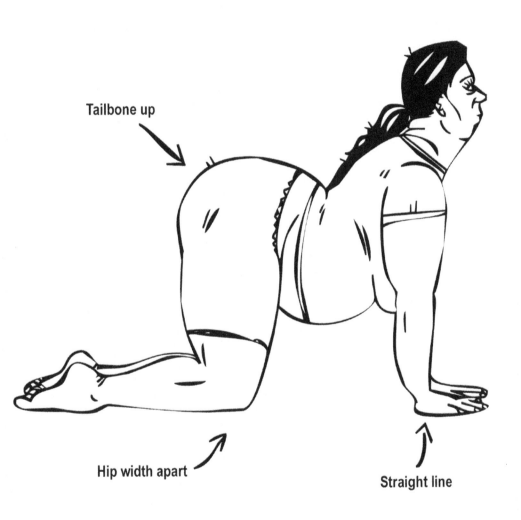

Tailbone up

Hip width apart

Straight line

9. Cat Pose – *Marjaryasana*

How to do it:

Hands and knees, table position, just like the last one. Now instead of going down, you round your spine towards the sky as you exhale. Release your head downwards but don't strain your neck. You're a cat now. Inhale and go back to being a table, or go down further to transform into a cow if you want all the fun. Repeat.

Why do it:

- Stretches back torso and neck.
- Massages the spine and belly organs.
- Cats are cooler than cows.

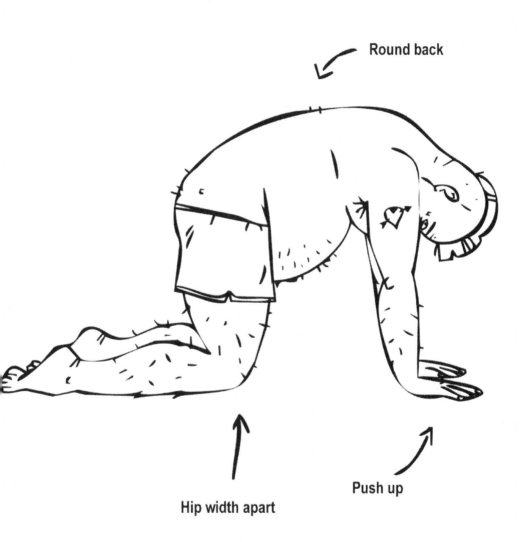

Round back

Push up

Hip width apart

10. Extended Puppy Pose – *Uttana Shishosana*

How to do it:

Next up is the **Puppy** pose, also known as the doggy position to regular people. You're going to be a pro at this. If you're still on all fours, good. Now walk the hands forward but keep your legs in position. Then lower down your head and torso. See if you can rest your forehead on the mat, or perhaps even your chest. Legs are still in position. Breathe in and out while sinking deep into the stretch.

Why do it:

- Stretches the spine and shoulders.
- Puppies.
- Multi-purpose.

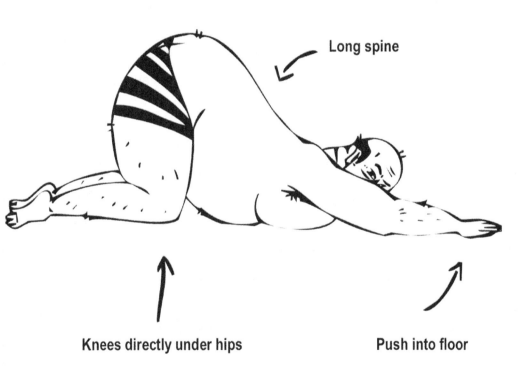

Long spine

Knees directly under hips

Push into floor

11. Downward Facing Dog – *Adho Mukha Svanasana*

How to do it:

When the puppy is ready to grow up, come onto your hands and knees again for this absolute classic. Tuck your toes under and lift your ass towards the sky. The feet are hip distance apart. Stretch your legs, press your thighs back and your hands into the mat for a long, straight back. Don't worry if your heels don't touch the mat, you'll get there eventually, maybe. Also spread your fingers. You now look like a triangle rather than a dog, but you can pretend to be whatever you like while you breathe in and out for five breaths.

Why do it:

- Strengthens arms and legs.
- Stretches shoulders, hamstrings, calves, arches of the feet, and hands.
- A rush of oxygen-rich blood to the head.

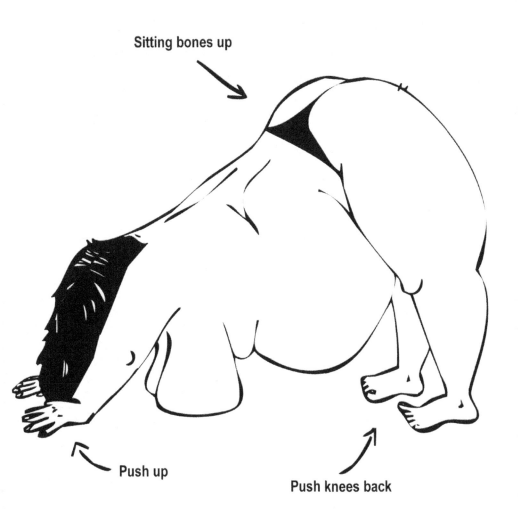

Sitting bones up

Push up

Push knees back

12. Plank Pose – *Phalakasana*

How to do it:

You probably know this one. You may start from your hands and knees, or from **Downward Facing Dog**. Wrists go directly under your shoulders, extend your arms and legs. Form a straight plank from your heels to the top of your head. Look to the floor and try not to let your hips sag. Hold, hold, hooooooold. And keep breathing. Seriously, this is a good pose to try and hold for a longer duration every time you do it. The more seconds, the more abs.

Why do it:

- Strengthens the arms, wrists, spine, and abdomen.
- Look at that six-pack.
- Abs.

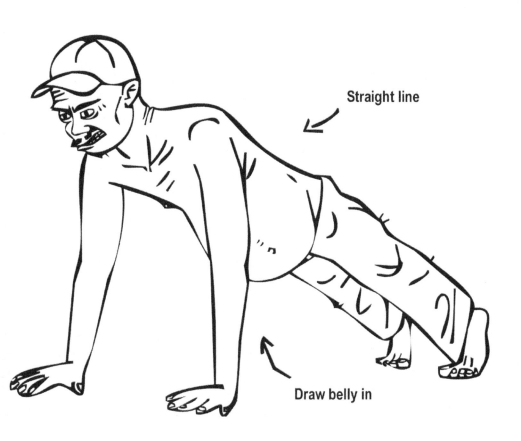

Straight line

Draw belly in

13. Four-Limbed Staff Pose – *Chaturanga Dandasana*

How to do it:

Another classic that is part of many sequences, such as the Sun Salutation. Usually, you start in **Downward Facing Dog**, move into **Plank** pose, and then lower down into **Four-Limbed Staff**. Lower down until your shoulders are at elbow height and keep your elbows close to the body. As with the **Plank**, your body forms a straight line and is engaged from the toes up. Gaze down, and again, don't let your hips sag. You want that chiseled set of rock-hard abs, don't you? Of course you do. Hold the pose for a couple breaths or for a couple minutes to really work those abs. Try not to use your belly for support, but if you can't help it, so be it.

Why do it:

- Strengthens arms and core.
- Gives you a chiseled set of rock-hard abs.
- You're a fabulous four-limbed staff.

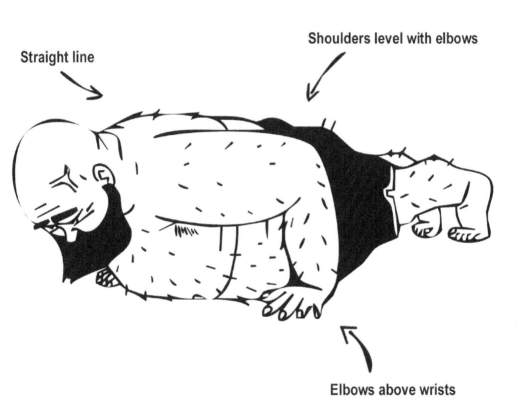

Straight line

Shoulders level with elbows

Elbows above wrists

14. Cobra Pose – *Bhujangasana*

How to do it:

If you're still holding the **Four-Limbed Staff**, good. If not, get back in position. Now exhale and lower the whole body down to the mat. Slowly, preferably. With the top of the feet on the mat you roll your shoulders back and keep the elbows close to the body. Now push yourself up with your arms, chest forward and leave your legs where you put them. Go up as far as is comfortable. You now look like a cobra, ready to strike. Or to dance. Depends on what kind of cobra you are.

Why do it:

- Strengthens spine.
- Stretches chest, shoulders, and abdomen.
- Awakens your kundalini, whatever that is.

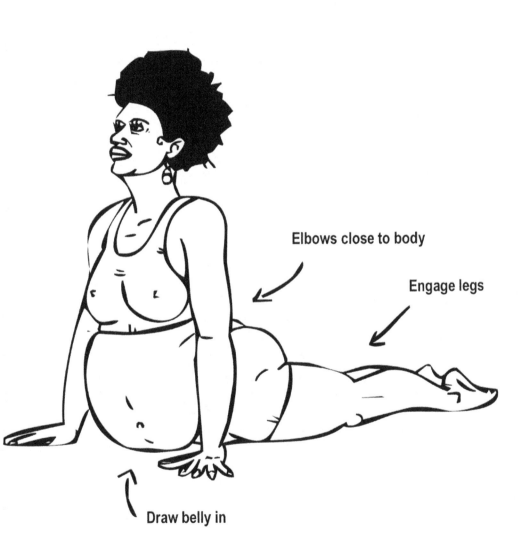

Elbows close to body

Engage legs

Draw belly in

15. Low Lunge Pose – *Anjaneyasana*

How to do it:

Get back into **Downward Facing Dog**. Step your right foot between your hands. Drop the left knee to the mat with the top of the foot on the mat. Make sure the forward knee points straight forward and is aligned with the heel. If you can keep your balance, raise your arms up and back and stare at your hands with a slight backbend. Otherwise you can stare at whatever is in front of you. The tv probably, or a pizza. Now sink your butt down for a good stretch of the groins and thighs. Switch legs and repeat.

Why do it:

- Stretches thighs and groins.
- Improves balance and leg strength.
- Opens the chest, not literally.

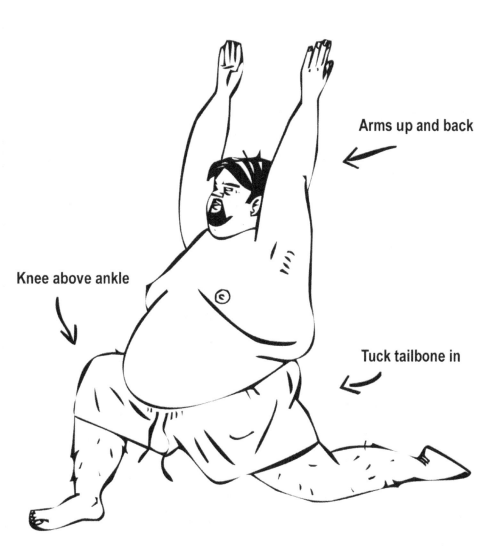

Arms up and back

Knee above ankle

Tuck tailbone in

16. Crescent Lunge Pose – *Ashta Chandrasana*

How to do it:

This one is similar to the **Low Lunge**, but we're going to make it a little harder because you love a good challenge. Start in **Low Lunge**, then tuck your toes and lift your back knee up from the floor, straighten your leg and that's it. Raise your arms over your head if you can, like the last pose. Now breathe in and out and try not to fall over. The deeper you go, the better the stretch, but don't hurt yourself. Keep the core engaged for stability. Five breaths and repeat on the other leg.

Why do it:

- Stretches the groins.
- Strengthens the legs and arms.
- Improves balance and leg strength.

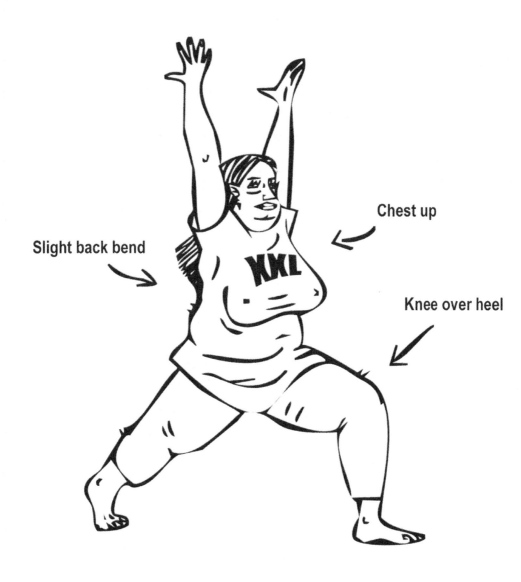

Slight back bend

Chest up

Knee over heel

17. Warrior I – *Virabhadrasana I*

How to do it:

Enough with the lame animals, we're going to pose like a proper warrior now. This is a variation of the last pose, difference being that you're no longer allowed to lift your heel off the mat. Instead, you turn your foot 45 degrees and keep your heel on the mat. Align the feet. If you want more stretch, place your feet wider apart. Hands in the sky as if you're shooting your kundalini pistols at the moon, being the warrior that you are.

Why do it:

- Stretches pretty much your whole body.
- Strengthens shoulders, arms, back and legs.
- You're a badass.

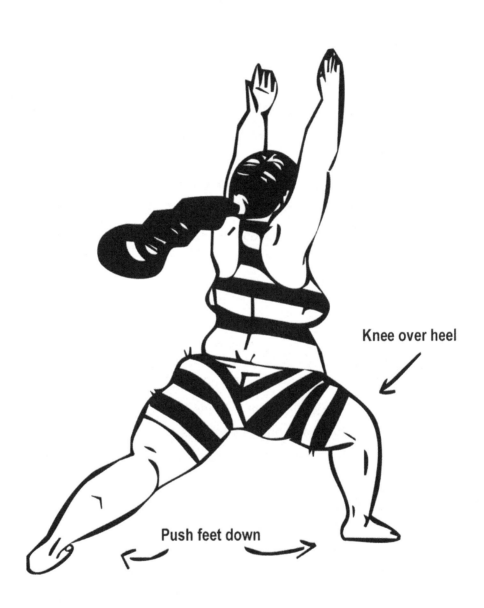

Knee over heel

Push feet down

18. Warrior II – *Virabhadrasana II*

How to do it:

Legs are in the same position as with **Warrior I**. Now instead of shooting your kundalini pistols in the air, imagine there's enemies both in front of you and behind you. Reach your arms out parallel to the mat, palms facing down. Face forward. Stand firm. This pose is named after an incarnation of Shiva, a fierce warrior with a thousand heads and a thousand eyes, so I guess all of his heads have only one eye. That's you now.

Why do it:

- Stretches ankles, legs, groin, and hips.
- Strengthens legs, abdominals, arms, and shoulders.
- A thousand one-eyed heads.

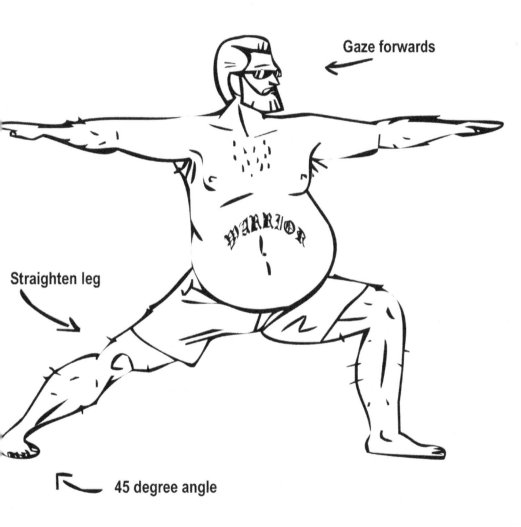

Gaze forwards

Straighten leg

45 degree angle

19. Standing Forward Bend – *Uttanasana*

How to do it:

We're taking a step back in coolness. We will see some very cool poses again, later on. For this one, start in **Mountain** pose, big toes touching. Exhale and bend forward from the hips with an open chest. Keep your legs straight if you can and see if you can touch your toes. Grab your big toes or place your hands flat on the mat if this is too easy. If you're stiff as hell or have T-Rex arms you can grab your shins instead. Deepen the pose slightly with each breath. Like the **Seated Forward Bend**, you can also do this one with legs wider apart.

Why do it:

- Stretches hamstrings, calves, and hips.
- Apparently stimulates the liver and kidneys (for you alcoholics).
- Maybe you can touch your toes someday.

Hinge from the hips

Straight legs

Relax neck

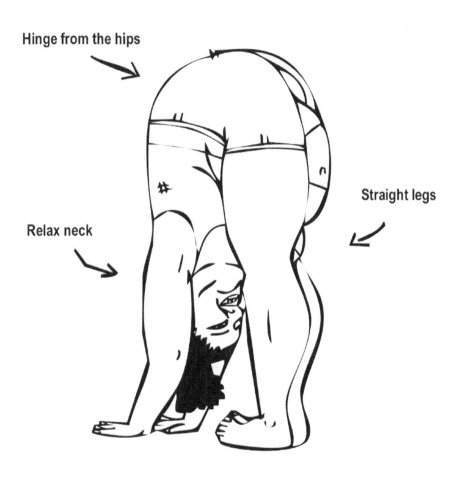

20. Chair Pose – *Utkatasana*

How to do it:

Get back to **Mountain** pose. Now slowly bend your knees and sit back and down while lifting your arms up. Engage your core and keep your chest open. Keep breathing and come back to **Mountain** pose when you're ready (that is, tired). Feel the burn in your quads. You may find that it's not that easy being a chair, but it is good for you. Keep all involved muscles engaged to prevent you from actually sitting down.

Why do it:

- Strengthens thighs, calves, ankles and spine.
- Reduces flat feet, how about that?
- Stretches shoulders and chest.

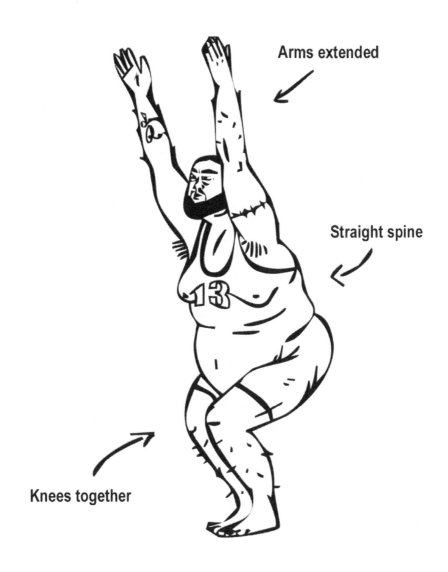

Arms extended

Straight spine

Knees together

21. Happy Baby Pose – *Ananda Balasana*

How to do it:

This one's easy and fun if your legs are tired from the last pose. Lie on your back and bring your knees into your belly. Lift your feet and grab them from the outside with your hands or grab your big toes, then bring your knees down and towards your armpits while opening your legs. Play around to find the best stretch and relax.

Why do it:

- Good excuse to act like a baby again.
- Stretches the groins and the back of the spine.
- Relaxing, don't fall asleep.

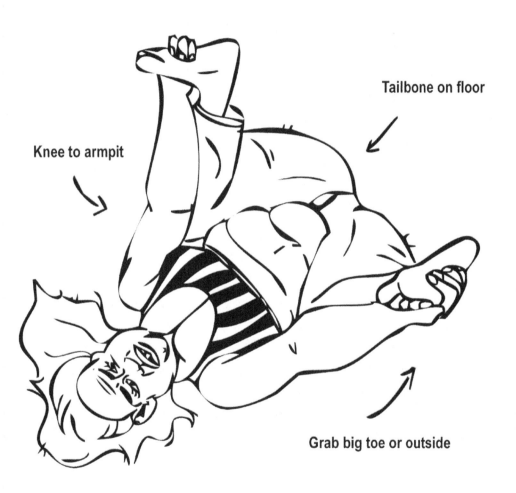

Tailbone on floor

Knee to armpit

Grab big toe or outside

22. Garland Pose – *Malasana*

How to do it:

This a great alternative for your regular office slouch, though your colleagues will probably laugh at you. Start in **Mountain** pose and step the feet hip-width apart with the toes pointing outward. Keep the heels on the mat while you lower down to a squatting position. You may push your hands together with your elbows against your knees to prevent you from slouching forward. Keep the chest open. Hold for five breaths or stay here and continue writing that assignment for your boss.

Why do it:

- Stretches ankles, groins and back torso.
- Improves posture.
- An alternative way of sitting that is healthier.

Chest up

Elbows press into knees

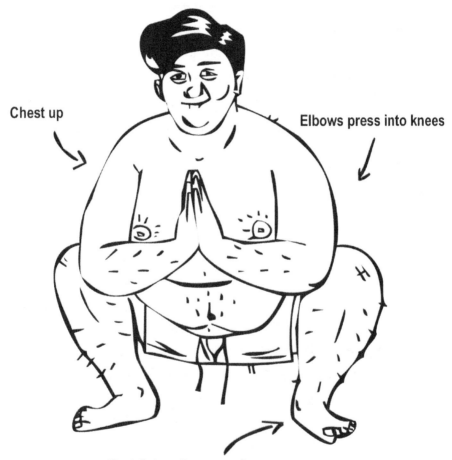

Feet flat on the ground

23. Tree Pose – *Vrksasana*

How to do it:

Get back up to **Mountain** pose, big toes touching. Then raise your knee and grab your foot or ankle. Place your foot against your thigh and gently press the thigh and foot against each other. Stand straight with your hands in your waist, in prayer position, or in the air. If you keep falling over, try it with the support of a wall first, and if you can't place your foot into your thigh, place it on your calf, not on the knee. Take a couple of deep breaths, chant some Oms and get back to **Mountain** pose. Repeat on the other leg.

Why do it:

- Strengthens thighs, calves, ankles.
- Improves balance.
- Stretches groins and inner thighs.

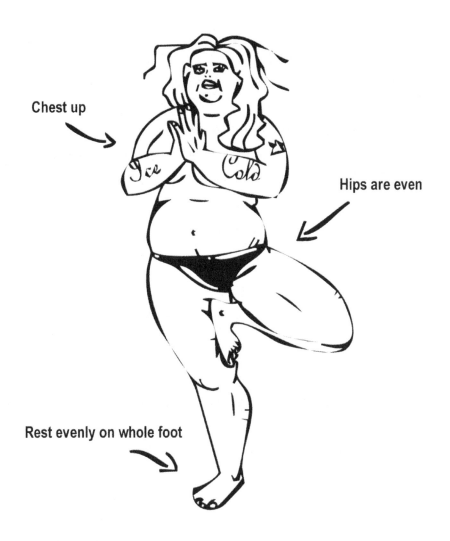

Chest up

Hips are even

Rest evenly on whole foot

24. Corpse Pose – *Savasana*

How to do it:

Some regard this pose as the hardest of them all. I'd say that's a little exaggerated. Relaxing may be hard for some, but any effort is good effort. As the name suggests, we will now be playing dead. Lie on your back with your feet slightly apart, arms next to your body. Palms up and let your feet fall to the sides. Breathe in and out, letting go of any tension in the body. Return your attention to the breath if you notice yourself getting distracted. Do this for 5 to 10 minutes for a relaxing end of your workout. It's also a good way to fall asleep so watch out, or sweet dreams.

Why do it:

- Total relaxation of mind and body.
- An exercise in meditation.
- Who doesn't love naps?

Concentrate on breath

Palms up

Close eyes

Chapter 2: The Advanced Yogi

Since you've made it this far, I'd say you can call yourself a yogi now. Tell your friends. Tell them about this book so they will buy it as well and become yogis too. We'll now be moving on to harder poses. Here's a vague inspirational quote to help you along:

> "Yoga is the journey of the self, through the self, to the self."
>
> – The Bhagavad Gita

25. Half Moon Pose – *Ardha Chandrasana*

How to do it:

Let's start this chapter with a tricky pose right off the bat. Start in **Warrior II**. Now slowly bend your upper body forward until your front arm touches the mat. Step your back leg forward a bit and place your front arm a little further as well. Straighten your front leg and lift your back leg into the air at the same time. Turn your chest upwards and extend your other arm into the sky. Adjust as needed at any point and use something to support your arm if you can't reach the mat without falling over. Switch sides.

Why do it:

- Improves coordination and balance.
- Strengthens abdomen, ankles, thighs, buttocks and back.
- Stretches groins, hamstrings, calves, shoulders, chest, and spine.

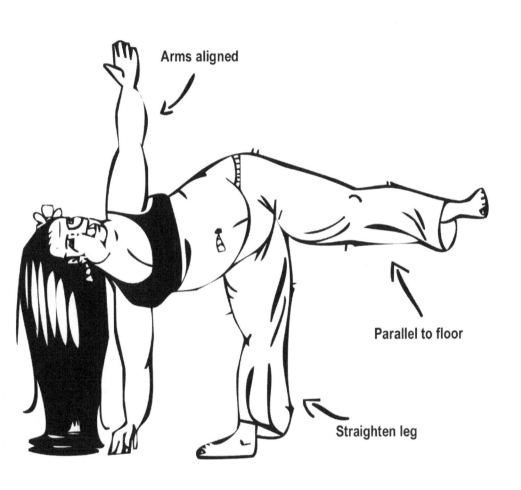

Arms aligned

Parallel to floor

Straighten leg

61

26. Warrior III Pose – *Virabhadrasana III*

How to do it:

The last and hardest of the warrior series. Start in **Mountain** pose and step your right leg forward, bending it slightly. Hands in the waist and back straight, then slowly shift your weight forward and raise your left leg in the air. Find your balance, then straighten your legs and straighten your arms forward. You can also reach your hands behind you for an airplane pose, or one fist to the front and the other to the side for the Super(wo)man pose. Hold, lower back down and repeat on the other leg.

Why do it:

- Strengthens the ankles, legs, shoulders, back and abs.
- Improves balance.
- Re-enact your favorite Superman scenes.

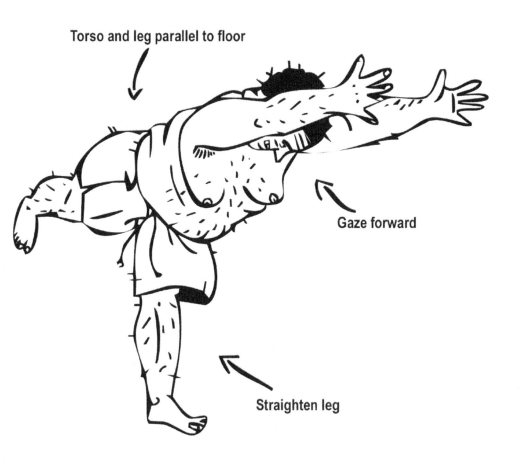

Torso and leg parallel to floor

Gaze forward

Straighten leg

27. Revolved Triangle Pose – *Parivrtta Trikonasana*

How to do it:

From **Mountain** pose, step your feet a meter apart and turn your right foot 90 degrees to the right and your left 45 degrees. Spread your arms to the side and twist your body to the right, but keep your feet planted and your legs straight, don't bend your knees. Now place your left hand on the mat, either on the inside, outside (better stretch) or on the ankle of the right foot. Twist your body further, extending your right arm to the sky. Keep the back straight and chest open at all times. Switch sides and do it again. You may place your hand on a support if you keep falling over otherwise.

Why do it:

- Stretches the legs, hips and spine.
- Improves balance.
- Good for a sore back.

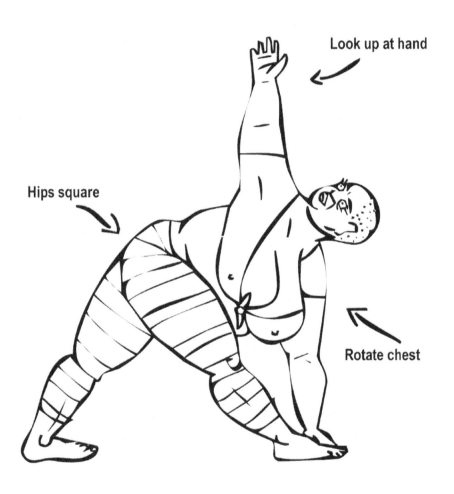

Look up at hand

Hips square

Rotate chest

65

28. Side plank pose – *Vasisthasana*

How to do it:

Relatively easy to get into, but pretty hard to hold for more than a couple seconds; the side plank. Start in **Plank** pose, then slowly roll over to your side, placing the left foot on top of the right and raising your left arm up to the sky so that you're now balancing on your right hand and foot. Keep your body straight like a plank. If you suck at this, try placing your left foot in front of your right for more balance. If you're feeling frisky, however, then try to straighten your left leg as high as you can. Hold for five or as long as you can and repeat on the other hand.

Why do it:

- Strengthens the wrists, arms, abs, and legs.
- Improves balance.
- Crazy side abs.

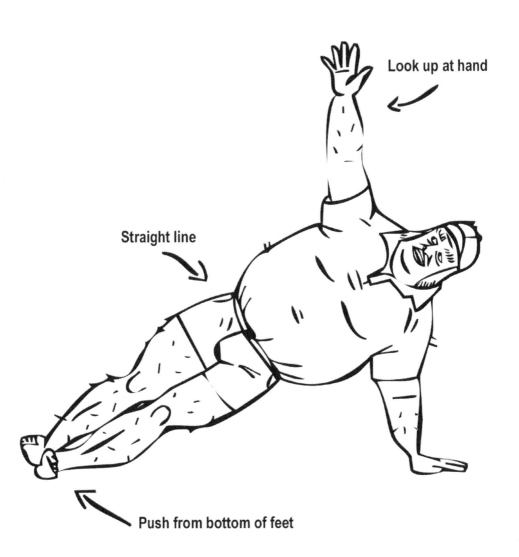

Look up at hand

Straight line

Push from bottom of feet

29. Eagle Pose – *Garudasana*

How to do it:

By now you're probably thinking 'Mothersmucker, bring back the easy peasy animal poses.' Well, there's good and bad news. The bad news is no more easy poses, the good news is that we've got many cool animals left in store. For the **Eagle** pose, you start in **Mountain** pose. Lift your right knee to your chest, then lower it down and wrap it around the left leg, bending the left knee slightly. Keep your balance while placing the right arm underneath the left upper arm and touch your palms together. Lift your elbows up for the full **Eagle**. Repeat on the other leg.

Why do it:

- Stretches thighs, hips, shoulders, upper back, ankles and calves.
- Improves balance and concentration.
- You're an apex predator for a minute.

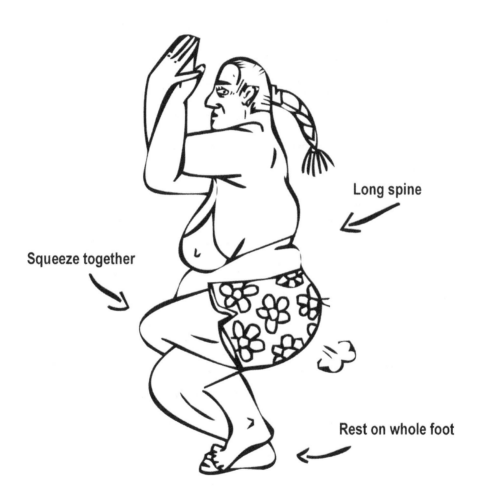

Long spine

Squeeze together

Rest on whole foot

30. Extended Hand-To-Big-Toe – *Utthita Hasta Padangustasana*

How to do it:

From **Mountain** pose you raise your right knee to the chest once more. Grab your big toe with your right index and middle finger and keep your elbow on the inside of your leg. The left hand is in the waist. Now slowly extend your heel away from you without falling over until your leg is completely straight. Repeat with the other leg. You can also shift your leg out to the side for an extra challenge. Wash your hands afterwards because they will smell like toes.

Why do it:

- Stretches the calves and back of the legs.
- Improves balance.
- Strengthens the legs as well as the index and middle fingers.

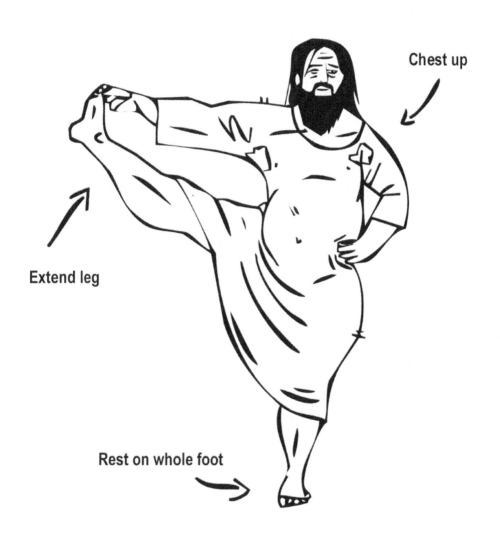

Chest up

Extend leg

Rest on whole foot

31. Camel Pose – *Ustrasana*

How to do it:

This is a good back bender that is a great counter for your office hunch and another absolutely glorious animal. Start by standing on your knees, place them slightly apart and place your hands on the top of your ass. Look up and push your hips forward while slowly arching your back. Go down until you can grab your heels and that's it. Make sure you warm up well before this one, especially if you're stiff as a board. Engage your core, don't let yourself just fall over or you might strain your back. Enjoy the stretch and come into **Child's** pose afterwards for a nice counter stretch.

Why do it:

- Good for your posture.
- Stretches the abs, chest, ankles, thighs and groins.
- Camels have three eyelids and two rows of eyelashes.

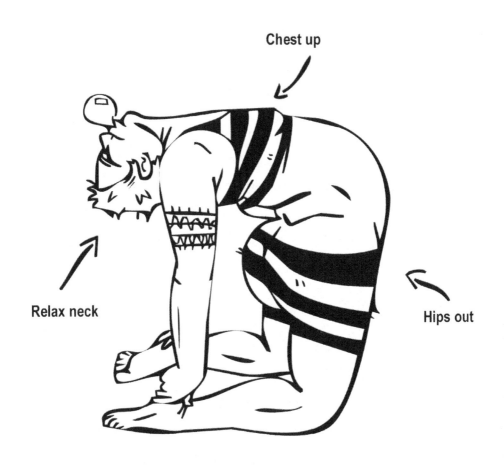

Chest up

Relax neck

Hips out

32. Bow Pose – *Dhanurasana*

How to do it:

This one is like the **Camel** pose, just rotated 90 degrees. But don't faceplant forward and think you got it. Begin by lying on your belly and grabbing the outsides of your feet or your ankles. Relax your butt muscles. Now inhale and lift up the torso and knees so that you're balancing on your belly. This might be one of the few poses that are easier for chubby people, so enjoy that fact. Push your legs upwards as far as you can, but don't let go of them. You can hold the pose for a couple breaths or slowly go up and down for a proper workout set.

Why do it:

- Good for your posture.
- Stretches the abs, chest, ankles, thighs and groins.
- Strengthens the back muscles.

Gaze straight

Shoulders drawn together

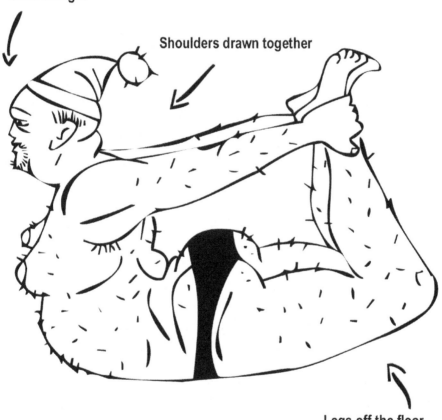

Legs off the floor

33. Wheel Pose – *Urdhva Dhanurasana*

How to do it:

Start by lying on the mat on your back and drawing your feet towards your ass, hip distance apart. Arms are on the mat alongside your body. It may be smart to warm up a little by bringing your hips up a couple times, raising as much of your torso off the mat as you can. Now for the real **Wheel**, you place your hands next to your head with your fingers pointing towards your feet. Keep your elbows in, lift your hips up again and push yourself up, extending the arms and legs as far as you can. Now do some reverse pushups if you can.

Why do it:

- Strengthens wrists, arms, legs, buttocks, abs and spine.
- Good for your posture.
- Walk around like this and you look like a mutant zombie.

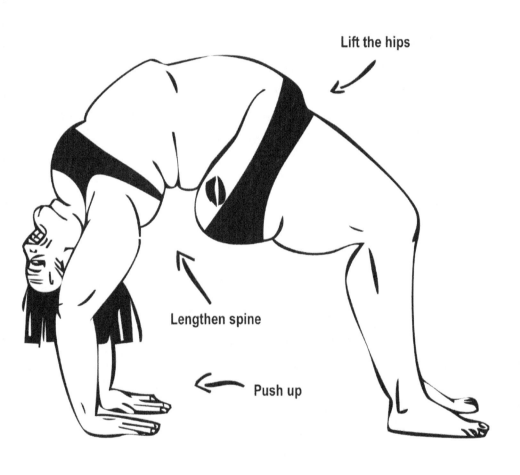

Lift the hips

Lengthen spine

Push up

34. Upward Plank Pose – *Purvottanasana*

How to do it:

Another reversal of a pose we've seen before, this time of the **Plank**. Start out in **Staff** pose. Place your hands behind you with the fingers still pointing towards the feet. Toes forward. Bend a little backwards and lift your hips off the ground until you're straight as a plank again. Also use your hands and feet to push yourself up. Chest up. Five breaths or hold for a minute or so.

Why do it:

- Strengthens the arms, wrists, legs, core and buttocks.
- Helps you open up to new possibilities.
- Another posture improver.

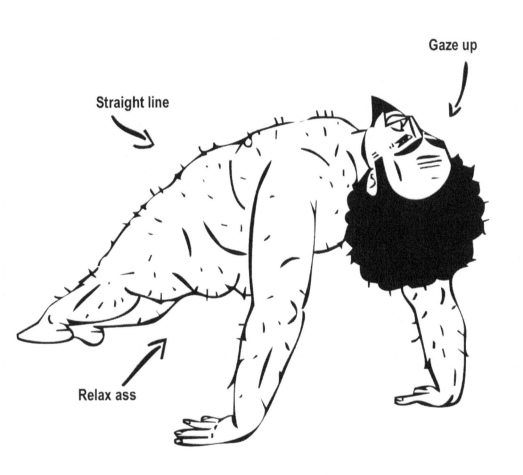

Gaze up

Straight line

Relax ass

35. Boat Pose – *Paripurna Navasana*

How to do it:

This one may look a little stupid, but it's a real ab killer and a good challenge. You're going to make a V shape and balance on your ass (tailbones). Start from a sitting position and lean back slightly while lifting your shins parallel to the floor. Straight back and chest up. Raise your arms in line with your shins and balance on your sitting bones. For the full pose, straighten your legs 45 degrees upwards and point your arms towards your feet, palms facing each other. Hold for a couple breaths to start and work your way to a minute without sinking.

Why do it:

- Strengthens abs, hip flexors and spine.
- Improves posture.
- Helps digest all the mess you're eating.

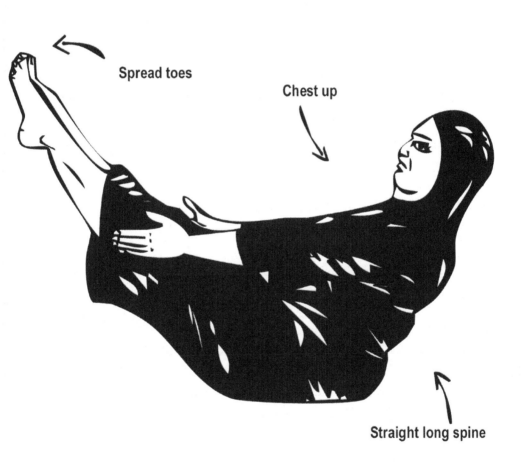

Spread toes

Chest up

Straight long spine

36. Plow Pose – *Halasana*

How to do it:

This one's fun and not even that hard. Maybe it should've been in the first chapter. Lie on your back, hands along your body with the palms down. Now raise the legs up and over your head but keep your hands where they are. Roll your legs all the way over until the toes touch the ground and straighten your legs. Straighten your back as well, don't round it too much. Use your hands for support. Keep your head facing forward, otherwise you risk straining your neck. Enjoy this weirdly pleasant position for a couple breaths and return. You can also lower your knees to your ears for an extra stretch.

Why do it:

- Weirdly calming.
- Stretches the shoulders and spine.
- Also helps for insomnia, infertility and a bunch of other stuff, or so they say.

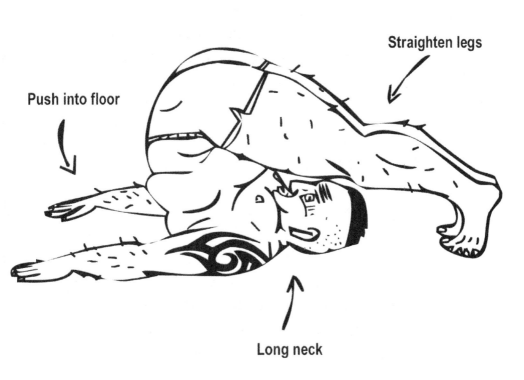

Straighten legs

Push into floor

Long neck

37. Marichi's Pose I – *Marichyasana I*

How to do it:

I don't know who **Marichi** is, but he's got a whopping eight yoga poses dedicated to him. We're not going to do all of them because they mostly work the same muscles and some of them are pretty outrageous (look up the last one). Anyway, for the first one, start by sitting in **Staff** pose and fold your left leg to your body with a bit of width between your left foot and right leg. Raise your arms up and chest out, then fold forward. Hook your left arm around your left knee towards the back and grab it with your right if you can. Now fold forward even more and rest your forehead on your shin. Switch sides.

Why do it:

- Stretches the spine and shoulders.
- Squeezes your internal organs (this is good).
- Helps against obesity and constipation (says tradition).

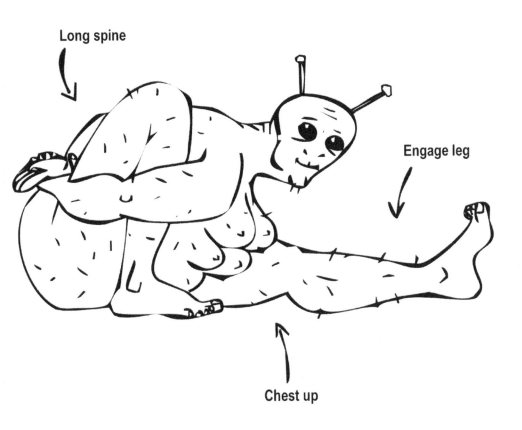

38. Marichi's Pose III – *Marichyasana III*

How to do it:

I just looked up **Marichi** and apparently, he was (or is?) the god-son of Brahma, the creator of pretty much everything. Marichi cursed his wife and turned her into a stone, but people still worship him. Start in **Staff** pose again and bring your right leg to your body. Straighten your back and open your chest. Wrap your left arm around your knee and grab it from the back with the other hand. If you're too stiff to connect you can use your right arm to support you instead. Twist your torso to the right and keep your left leg active, toes up. Deepen the twist with each inhale. Release slowly and switch sides.

Why do it:

- Stretches and strengthens the spine and shoulders.
- A nice massage for your belly organs.
- A good brain stimulator, apparently.

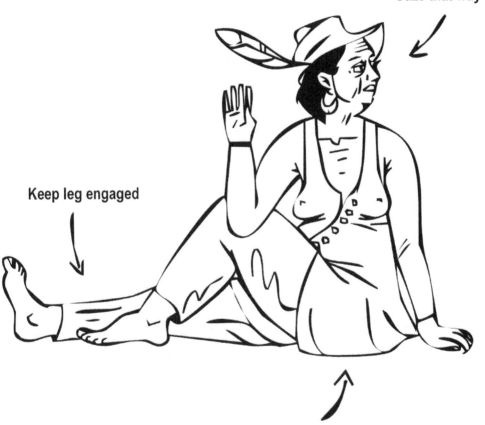

39. Upward Facing Dog Pose – *Urdhva Mukha Svanasana*

How to do it:

The counter to the classic. Start in **Downward Facing Dog**, shift your body forward into **Plank** pose but place the top of your feet on the mat instead of the toes. Sink your body down, but keep your arms straight or slightly bent, chest forward and draw your shoulder blades toward each other. Use both legs and arms. Didn't we do this already? Nope, this one's similar to the **Cobra** pose, but in this one you're not supposed to touch the mat with anything but hands and feet. The time to relax is long over, friends.

Why do it:

- Strengthens the back, arms, wrists and booty.
- Stretches chest, shoulders and abs.
- Another pose that improves posture.

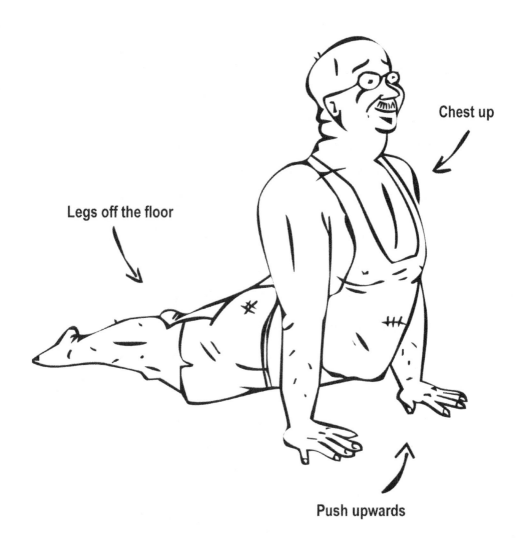

40. Monkey Pose – *Hanumanasana*

How to do it:

People always ask me who would win in battle, Hanuman, leader of the mythological monkey army, or Saruman, leader of orcs? All I'm going to say is that I haven't seen Saruman flying through the air doing splits, which is what Hanuman is famous for. This pose is dedicated to Hanuman. Try this only when you're ready, that is, when you are flexible enough to do the **Lunges** and **Forward Bends** without trouble. Starting on hands and knees, you step the right foot forward between your hands. Slide the left knee back and slowly crawl the right foot more and more forward. Keep the hips square and use something for support while easing into the pose if needed (tip: yoga block, brick, chair). Finish it off with your hands in the sky. Switch legs and do it again.

Why do it:

- Stretches the thighs, hamstrings, groins.
- You will be flexible enough to kick people in the head.
- Stimulates the digestive and reproductive organs.

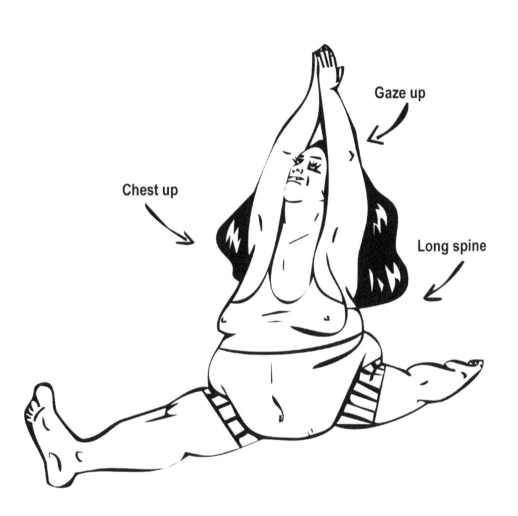

41. Supported Shoulder Stand – *Salamba Sarvangasana*

How to do it:

Lie down on your back and bring your knees to your chest. Arms are alongside your body and press into the mat to help you lift your hips from the mat. Work your core and keep your knees bent but don't knee yourself in the face. Place your hands on your back for support and walk them down to prop your torso up as straight as possible. Finally, raise your knees up and extend your legs straight up towards the sky. Beautiful. Hold for at least five breaths.

Why do it:

- Strengthens the abs, legs, buttocks.
- Stretches shoulders and neck.
- A nice rush of oxygen-rich blood to the head.

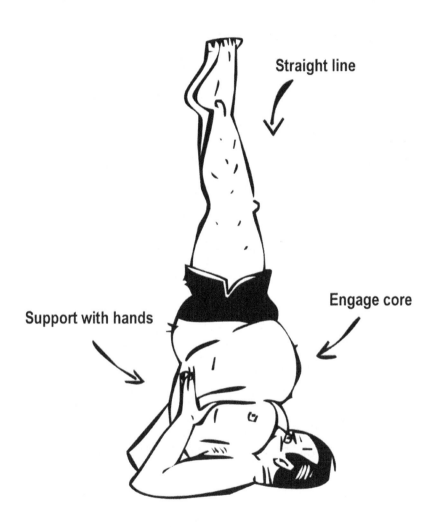

Straight line

Engage core

Support with hands

93

42. Supported Headstand – *Salamba Sirsasana*

How to do it:

We're going one step further for this one. Start on all fours, but now on your knees and elbows. Grab your elbows with your hands to get the right distance between them. Then move your hands forward and interlace your fingers where your hands meet. Place the top of the head on the ground and into your palms. Now stand your legs up and slowly walk them towards you. Bend one knee up into your chest, then the next. You are now in the air. Slowly raise your legs up to the sky until you're fully extended. Use your core strength for balance. If you happen to fall over backwards, tuck your chin to your chest so you don't break your neck. Happy practicing.

Why do it:

- Supposedly aids the production of sex hormones.
- Lots of oxygen to the brain.
- Strengthens arms, legs, back, abs, pretty much everything.

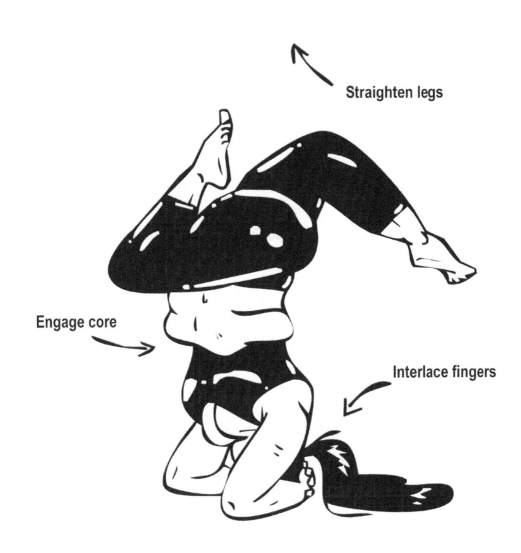

Straighten legs

Engage core

Interlace fingers

43. Crane/Crow Pose – *Bakasana*

How to do it:

This one's called the **Crane** (with straightened arms) or the **Crow** (bent arms) pose. Those birds don't look alike at all. It's also the last of the intermediate poses, after mastering this one you will be a true intermediate yogi. Start in a squat and bury your knees into your armpits. Shift forward until you're up on your toes and on your hands. Try and pull one foot off the mat and then the other. Use your mighty core for balance. You're now standing on your hands, who would've thought this to be possible? Hold for five breaths.

Why do it:

- Crazy arm and wrist strength, also works the abs.
- Stretches the back and the groins.
- You're doing handstands now.

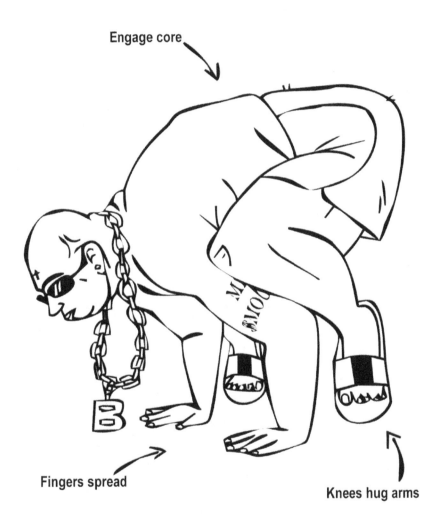

Engage core

Fingers spread

Knees hug arms

Chapter 3: The Yoga Master

Welcome to the last stage of your training, young Padawan. You have mastered many poses and overcome many challenges, but before you are a true Master, you will have to learn the poses in this chapter. Ignore the following quote:

"You must unlearn what you have learned."

– Yoda

44. Lotus Pose – *Padmasana*

How to do it:

This doesn't look hard and it isn't, the problem is just that you need crazy flexibility to pull it off. So warm up well and don't hurt your knees. Start in **Staff** pose, then bend your right leg at the knee and lift your foot onto the left thigh, sole facing up. Do the same with your other leg, lifting your foot onto your right thigh. Keep your back straight at all times. You may finally place your hands on your knees or in prayer position to attain full enlightenment.

Why do it:

- If Buddha got enlightened sitting like this, so can you.
- Stretches ankles and knees.
- Tradition says this pose heals disease and awakens your kundalini.

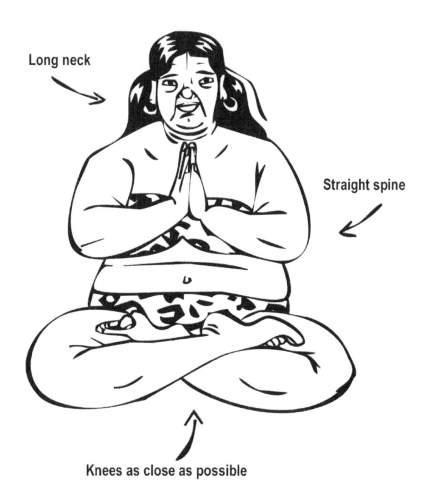

Long neck

Straight spine

Knees as close as possible

45. Firefly Pose – *Tittibhasana*

How to do it:

Let us do the Tittibhasana. Start in **Mountain** pose with your feet shoulder width apart and bend forward. The trick is to place your shoulders (or back of your arms) behind the calves, so bend your knees as needed and go one at a time. Once you're there, step your feet a little closer. Bend your knees while you place your palms on the ground behind your feet and lower that ass down. Slowly go from standing on all fours to balancing on your hands. Then, for the full pose, extend your legs fully.

Why do it:

- Stretches the groin, torso, legs.
- Arm and wrist strength.
- Improves balance.

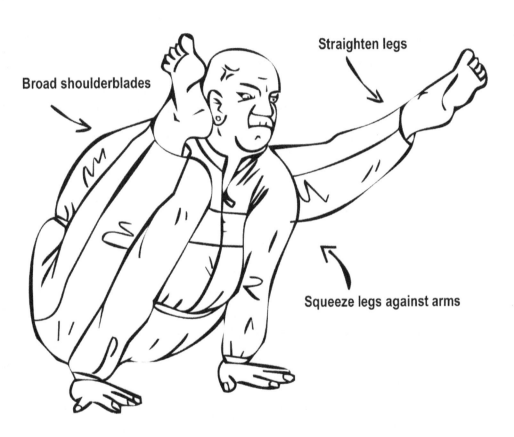

Broad shoulderblades

Straighten legs

Squeeze legs against arms

46. Lord of the Dance – *Natarajasana*

How to do it:

No joke, it's really called **Lord of the Dance**. With this pose you can combine much of what you've learned into a single pose. Start in Mountain pose, bend your right knee and grab the big toe side with your right hand. Keep the knees together, don't open the hips by going sideways. Reach forward with your left hand while you bend forward slowly, kicking the leg up as you go. Keep going until it looks like the picture on the right. Breathe in, breathe out. Release the leg and switch sides.

Why do it:

- Stretches most of your body.
- Strengthens legs and ankles.
- Dance move?

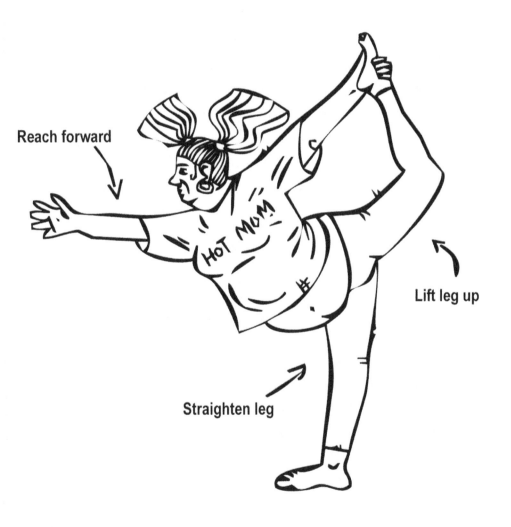

47. King Pidgeon Pose – *Kapotasana*

How to do it:

This pose is not for ordinary mortals. Try this only when you've mastered all the other backbends, or you might wreck yo self. Start by standing on your knees with your hands in prayer position. Slowly lower your torso down backwards. Let gravity do the work, but don't just drop down. When you're close enough to the mat you can stretch out the arms and let them find the mat, fingers pointing towards your feet. Now you're slowly going to walk your hands towards your feet, and if you get there, you place them on your heels. Keep your elbows close, not pointing out, and lower them down onto the ground.

Why do it:

- Stretches most of your body, especially the front.
- Strengthens the back.
- You have now mastered the flexibility skill.

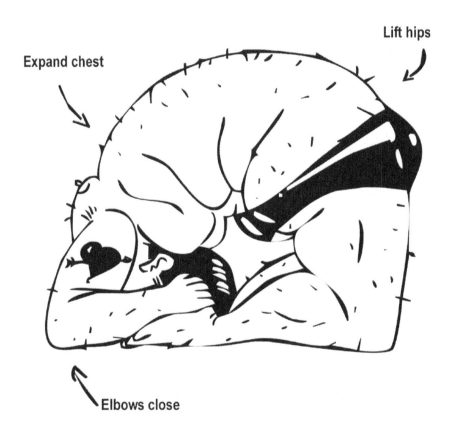

48. Peacock Pose – *Mayurasana*

How to do it:

Is it a handstand? Is it a plank? No, it's a **Peacock**. Do peacocks balance their whole bodyweight on their elbows? I don't know, but you will (after crashing to the mat a couple times, probably). Start by standing on your knees and bringing the arms to the body with the elbows in and fingers pointing down. Lower down your torso until your hands rest on the mat with the fingers pointing to your toes. Bend your elbows and bring them as close to each other as possible. Lean forward and lift the feet off the ground. Straighten your legs for the full pose and hold.

Why do it:

- Strengthens the wrists, arms, core, legs, torso.
- Improves balance.
- You can now impress those calisthenics bros.

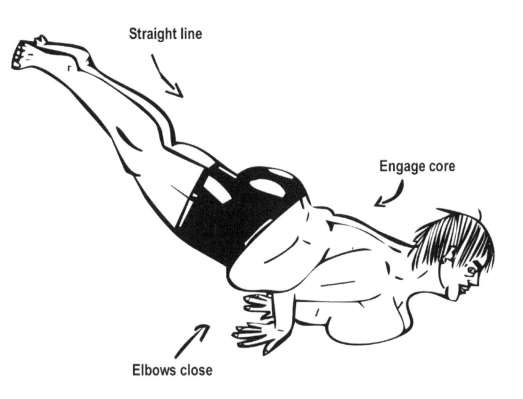

Straight line

Engage core

Elbows close

49. Shoulder Pressing Pose – *Bhujapidasana*

How to do it:

Similar to the **Firefly** pose, but perhaps slightly easier. No, the order of poses in this book does not make complete sense. The start is pretty much the same though; do that trick where you work your shoulders behind your calves from a forward bending position. Place your hands behind your feet, shoulder-width apart, and sink your ass down slowly. Lift your legs up off the mat and use your arms to push you up too. If you haven't fallen on your butt yet, cross your ankles.

Why do it:

- Strengthens shoulders, arms and wrists.
- Good ab workout.
- Improves balance.

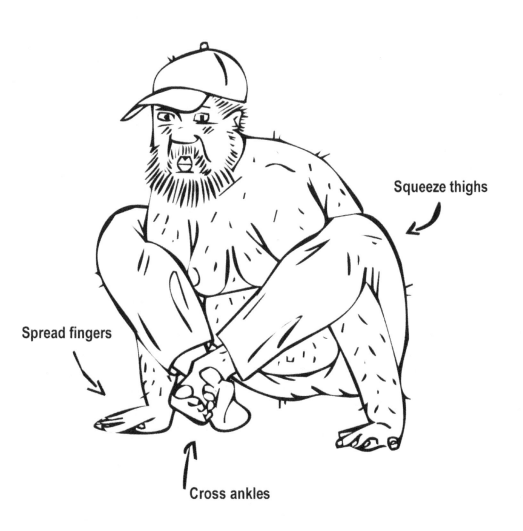

Squeeze thighs

Spread fingers

Cross ankles

50. Upward Facing Two Foot Staff – *Dwi Pada Viparita Dandasana*

How to do it:

Try this only when you can do the **Wheel** pose without effort. Start by doing the **Wheel** pose, then bend your arms and place your forearms on the mat with your elbows shoulder-width apart. Interlace your fingers and place the crown of your head into your hands. Now that you're standing on your head and forearms, you can slowly walk your feet forward (not towards your head) until your legs are fully extended. Look at that. To come out of the pose, get back to **Wheel** pose first.

Why do it:

- Improves your posture.
- Stretches and strengthens the whole front of your body.
- Opens the heart chakra to an advanced level, whatever that means.

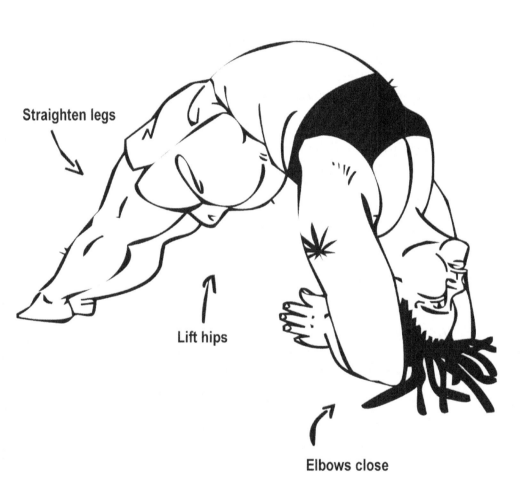

Straighten legs

Lift hips

Elbows close

51. Formidable Face Pose – *Ganda Bherundasana*

How to do it:

I have seen people do this, it really is physically possible. For a select few. Start on your belly with your chin on the mat. Slowly lift the legs up and over your head, arching the back. You probably need to use your arms for support. Bring the feet down next to or slightly in front of your face and grab them with your hands. Plant them on the ground and keep them there with your hands. Drape the forearms over your feet and rest your chin on your fingers. It's that easy. If you can do this and you also have a big enough butt, you can rest that butt right on top of your head. Formidable.

Why do it:

- 56/60 on the Iyengar difficulty scale (near-impossible).
- Stretches and strengthens the whole front of your body.
- Rest your butt on your head.

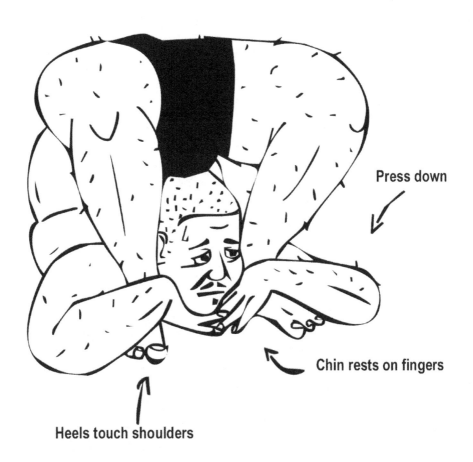

Press down

Chin rests on fingers

Heels touch shoulders

52. Handstand – *Adho Mukha Vrksasana*

How to do it:

For the final pose of this book we're going back to basics and then flip those basics upside down. You know, it's basically an inverted **Mountain** pose. There are multiple ways to do this. You can start in **Crow** pose and just reach out and up with your legs while keeping your balance. This requires a strong core and is definitely easier said than done. You can also start from **Downward Facing Dog** and walk your legs forward as far as you can. Start jumping one leg all the way up and come down, then do two. Keep your legs in whatever position you need to keep your balance. Then straighten your legs if you're ready. You can use a wall to practice. Now take a walk on your hands, Yogi Master.

Why do it:

- The ultimate balance improver.
- Strengthens core, legs, shoulders, arms, and wrists.
- Extra blood flow to the brain will boost your mood.

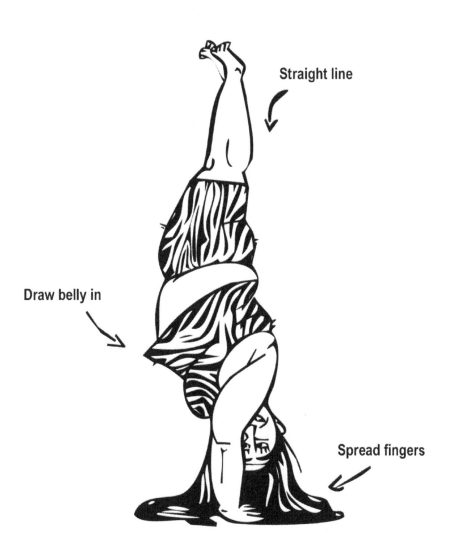

Straight line

Draw belly in

Spread fingers

Chapter 4: Here's Some Workouts

Now that you've mastered over 50 poses, you can create a personal little morning routine, or your own insane in the brain backbend campaign, whatever. But let's be honest, chances are you could use a little inspiration. This chapter gives you just that, in the form of four entry-level sequences. Feel free to mix and match, and don't forget:

"Each of us is a lake of love, yet strangely enough, we are all thirsty."

– Swami Kripalu

1. Saluting the Sun

The Sun Salutation, the most well-known yoga sequence. Great sequence to start your day or to warm up before a workout, as it stretches and strengthens the whole body. You can also do multiple repetitions to turn this sequence into a proper workout. Try starting with 5 minutes of repetitions and work your way up, and switch legs after every repetition. You can do this quickly or slowly. If you take it slow, take five breaths in every pose. If you want to go fast, then move into the next pose each time you inhale or exhale.

1. Start in **Mountain** pose and raise your arms to the sky. Gaze up towards your hands.
2. Fold into a **Standing Forward Bend**, then raise your torso up such that it is parallel to the floor with a straight spine.
3. Step back into a **Low** or **Crescent Lunge**.
4. Place your hands onto the mat and transition into **Downward Facing Dog**.
5. Lower down and forward into a **Plank**.
6. Lover down further into a **Four-Limbed Staff** pose.
7. Move into an **Upward Facing Dog**, **Cobra**, or **Sphinx** pose, depending on your skill and strength.
8. Do the sequence in reverse order until you end up in **Mountain** pose again.
9. That's it, champ.

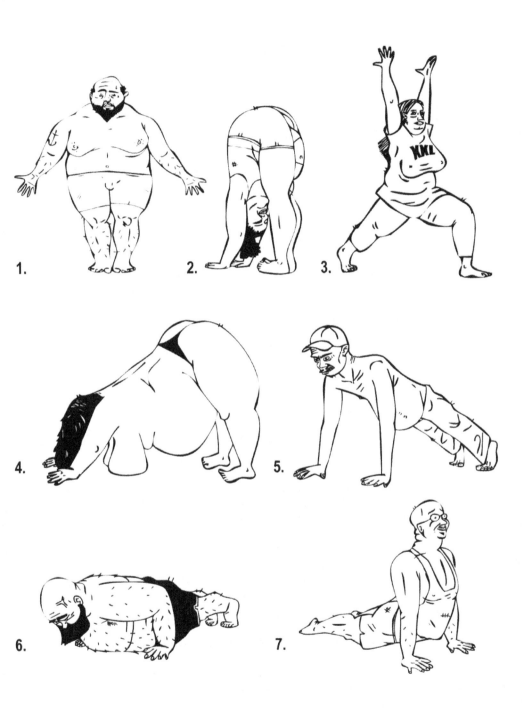

1.

2.

3.

4.

5.

6.

7.

2. Getting Flexible as a Rubber Band

Usually, your back is stiff as a board at the end of the day, but today is your lucky day. This sequence will flexibilize your body and mind, but mostly your body. It will also alleviate that back pain you get from sitting all day, so you can go back to the office and put in work with a smile. Your colleagues will wonder what happened to you, and they'll speculate behind your back. "Has she won the lottery?" "Did his mail-order bride arrive?" The only one who knows for sure is you. Since the main goal here is flexibility, it's important to really breathe into the pose, getting a deeper and deeper stretch with each breath.

1. Start in **Upward Dog**, or **Cobra**, or **Sphinx**.
2. Move up into **Downward Dog**.
3. Get into a **Seated Forward Bend**. You can vary with the **Wide-Angle Seated Forward Bend.**
4. Do a **Low** or **Crescent Lunge** to stretch the thighs.
5. Get on all fours and do the **Cat** pose.
6. Then do the **Cow** pose. Alternate Cat and Cow to relieve any tension in the back.
7. Do a **Bow** or **Camel** pose, or try the **Wheel** or **King Pidgeon** if you really want a challenge.
8. Finish stretching by moving into **Child's** pose.
9. You are now flexible enough to have your head up your ass both figuratively and literally.

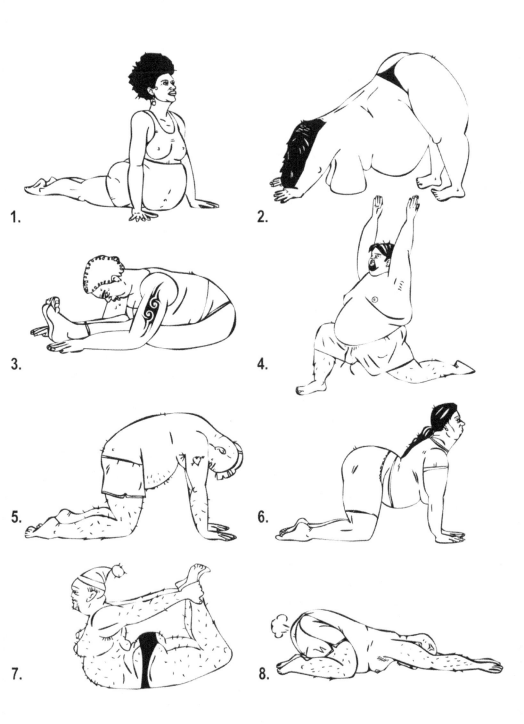

1.

2.

3.

4.

5.

6.

7.

8.

3. Abs You'd Kill For

If you've been living the yoga life for a while, then you probably have some notable ab development going on under that chubby coat, but maybe you'd rather have abs like Zack Efron in that one movie. Well, this sequence is designed to work your core from all angles, so that you too can get a chiseled set of rock-hard abs. It starts easy and gets harder as you go along, so if you can't do all the poses, just do the ones you can. I suggest you try to hold each pose for 30 seconds, then increase this every time you do the workout. Good luck, and don't forget to skip McDonalds every once in a while too.

1. Start in **Sphinx**, **Cobra** or **Upward Dog** for a good stretch of the front torso.
2. Get into a **Plank** pose and hold it.
3. Do the **Side Plank,** both sides.
4. Get back into a **Plank** and lower down into a **Four-Limbed Staff** pose.
5. Transition into **Warrior 3**. Switch legs.
6. Sit down and do a **Boat pose.** Bend your knees if you can't do the full pose right away.
7. Do the **Crow** pose, or one of the harder arm balances.
8. **Supported Shoulder** or **Head Stand** for core strength and balance.
9. Finish with the **Peacock** pose.
10. Go to the beach and show off those abs.

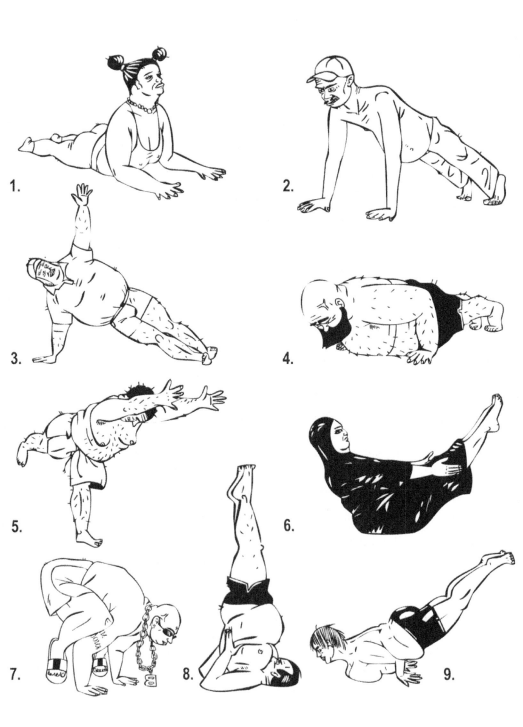

1.

2.

3.

4.

5.

6.

7.

8.

9.

125

4. The Chubby Yogi Relaxation Special

Yoga, like life itself, is not always about putting in effort. This sequence is for calming down and relaxing, as well as gently stretching the whole body. A great routine to do before going to bed after a long day, or before that afternoon nap, or any time, really. When the goal is to relax, don't push yourself as you might do normally, so work within a comfy range and breathe long and deep breaths. Take at least five breaths for every pose, but feel free to do more. Pro tip: you can do all of these in your bed and in your pajamas.

1. Start with a **Seated Forward Bend.**
2. Get on your belly and do the **Sphinx**.
3. Shift your buttocks back and do the **Extended Puppy**.
4. Step your knees a bit wider apart and sink into **Child's** pose.
5. Roll onto your back for the **Happy Baby** pose.
6. I find the **Plow** pose pleasantly calming, but skip this one if you disagree or find it hard to pull off.
7. Roll back into a sitting position for the **Easy** or **Lotus** pose. You can add in some meditation here if you're into that.
8. The one pose to rule them all, the **Corpse** pose. You can do this one under the blankets and until you fall asleep.
9. Sleep like a corpse. Sweet dreams.

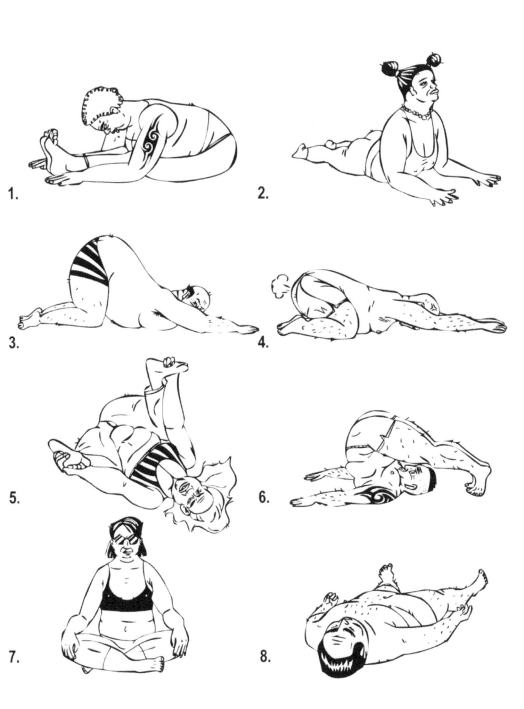

1.

2.

3.

4.

5.

6.

7.

8.

Epilogue

Congratulations, yogi. You have made it to the end of this book. You have mastered more than 50 mind and body-bending poses on your way to becoming a Yoga Master. You salute the sun daily. You live and breathe and sweat yoga. Now that you are enlightened, all that remains for you to do is travel the world and spread the message, teaching the world how to do the Adho Mukha Svanasana and the Tittibhasana. Tell the mortals to buy this book and bring the earth closer to world peace, one sale at a time. Paradise is upon us, let's do it together. Namaste.

Made in the USA
Coppell, TX
17 June 2020